Healing Earth:

A guide to medicinal herbs

By Tara Rowell

Contents

Introduction

In the bustling chaos of modern life, the quest for healing often leads us back to nature. Medicinal herbs, with their potent properties and centuries-old wisdom, offer a path to wellness that reconnects us with the earth's abundant gifts. "Healing Earth: A Guide to Medicinal Herbs" is a journey into the world of plant medicine, a comprehensive exploration of the healing power that lies within the leaves, roots, and flowers that surround us.

Chapter 1

The Wisdom of Herbal Medicine

The history of herbal medicine is as ancient as humanity itself, rooted in the earliest civilizations where people relied on the natural world for sustenance and healing. The origins of herbal medicine can be traced back to multiple cultures and civilizations across the globe, each contributing its unique knowledge and practices.

1. **Ancient Mesopotamia (Sumerians and Babylonians)**:

   The Sumerians and Babylonians, among the earliest civilizations, left behind written records of their use of herbs for medicinal purposes. Clay tablets dating back to around 2500 BCE contain lists of plants and their therapeutic properties. They used herbs like licorice, mustard, and thyme for various ailments.

2. **Ancient Egypt**:

   Ancient Egyptians are renowned for their advanced medical knowledge, which included the use of herbs. The Ebers Papyrus, one of the oldest medical texts dating back to around 1550 BCE, documents over 700 herbal remedies. Herbs like aloe vera, garlic, and coriander were commonly used for treating wounds, digestive issues, and other health problems.

3. **Ancient Greece**:

   Greek civilization made significant contributions to herbal medicine through figures like Hippocrates, often referred to as the "Father of Medicine." Hippocrates emphasized the importance of observing nature and the patient's symptoms in diagnosis and treatment. Greek physicians like Dioscorides compiled extensive herbal manuals, such as "De Materia Medica," which remained influential for centuries.

4. **Ancient China**:

   Traditional Chinese Medicine (TCM) has a history spanning thousands of years, with roots in ancient shamanic practices. The Huangdi Neijing (Yellow Emperor's Inner Canon), believed to have been written around 200 BCE, is a foundational text that emphasizes the balance of Yin and Yang and the use of herbs to restore harmony in the body. Chinese herbal medicine utilizes a vast array of plants, minerals, and animal products, with formulations often tailored to individual patients.

5. **Ayurveda (Ancient India)**:

   Ayurveda, the traditional medical system of India, dates back over 5,000 years. The ancient texts of Ayurveda, including the Charaka Samhita and Sushruta Samhita, detail the use of herbs and natural substances for promoting health and treating diseases. Ayurvedic medicine categorizes herbs based on their tastes (such as bitter, sweet, or pungent) and their effects on the body's doshas (bioenergetic forces).

These ancient civilizations discovered the healing properties of plants through a combination of trial and error, careful observation of nature, and intuitive wisdom passed down through generations. Herbal medicine was integral to their holistic approach to health, addressing not only physical symptoms but also the spiritual and emotional well-being of individuals.

Throughout history, the knowledge of medicinal herbs has been transmitted orally, through written texts, and through the apprenticeship of healers and shamans. Today, while modern medicine has made significant advancements, herbal medicine continues to thrive as people rediscover the benefits of natural remedies and seek alternatives to synthetic drugs.

Herbal medicine is a fascinating field that blends traditional knowledge with modern scientific understanding. Here's an exploration of the scientific principles underpinning herbal medicine:

1. **Phytochemistry**: This branch of chemistry deals with the study of plant-derived chemicals. Plants contain numerous bioactive compounds such as alkaloids, flavonoids, terpenoids, and phenolic compounds. These compounds are responsible for the therapeutic effects of herbs. Phytochemical analysis helps in identifying and characterizing these active constituents.

2. **Pharmacognosy**: Pharmacognosy is the study of medicinal drugs derived from natural sources, primarily plants. It involves identifying, selecting, and processing plant materials for medicinal use. Understanding the chemical composition of herbs helps pharmacognosists determine their therapeutic potential and safety profile.

3. **Pharmacology**: Pharmacology focuses on how drugs interact with biological systems. In herbal medicine, pharmacological studies investigate the mechanisms of action of plant compounds on various physiological processes. This includes studying their effects on receptors, enzymes, and signaling pathways in the body.

4. **Bioavailability**: Bioavailability refers to the proportion of a drug or compound that enters the bloodstream when introduced

into the body and is available for therapeutic action. Herbal medicines often contain complex mixtures of compounds that may influence their bioavailability. Factors such as absorption, metabolism, and distribution play crucial roles in determining the bioavailability of herbal constituents.

5. **Synergy and Multi-Compound Effects**: Herbal remedies often contain multiple bioactive compounds that can interact synergistically to produce enhanced therapeutic effects. This synergy is evident in traditional herbal formulations where different herbs are combined to create balanced remedies. Modern research aims to elucidate the synergistic interactions between plant compounds and understand how they contribute to the overall efficacy of herbal medicines.

6. **Target Identification**: Identifying molecular targets for herbal compounds is essential for understanding their mechanisms of action. Through techniques such as molecular docking, researchers can predict the binding affinity of plant compounds to specific receptors or enzymes implicated in disease processes. This knowledge aids in the development of targeted herbal therapies.

7. **Clinical Studies**: While traditional knowledge forms the basis of herbal medicine, modern clinical research provides scientific validation of its efficacy and safety. Clinical trials evaluate the effectiveness of herbal remedies in treating various conditions and compare them to standard treatments. Rigorous clinical studies help establish evidence-based guidelines for the use of herbal medicines in healthcare.

8. **Quality Control and Standardization**: Ensuring the quality and consistency of herbal products is crucial for their safety and efficacy. Quality control measures involve assessing the identity, purity, and potency of herbal preparations. Standardization techniques aim to establish uniformity in the composition of herbal products, allowing for reliable dosing and reproducible therapeutic effects.

By integrating these scientific principles, researchers can unravel the complex mechanisms of herbal medicine and harness the therapeutic potential of plant-based remedies for promoting health and wellness.

Chapter 3: Cultivating a healing garden

Growing your own medicinal herbs is not just about cultivating plants; it's about nurturing a connection with nature and harnessing its healing power. Let's embark on this journey together, shall we?

Planning Your Herbal Garden:

Start by selecting the herbs you want to grow based on your needs and climate. Consider factors like sunlight, soil type, and available space. Sketch out your garden layout, keeping in mind the growth habits and spacing requirements of each herb.

Planting Your Herbs:

Prepare the soil by enriching it with organic matter and ensuring proper drainage. Plant your herbs according to their specific needs, spacing them appropriately to allow for growth. Remember to label each herb to avoid confusion later on.

Caring for Your Garden:

Regular watering, weeding, and mulching are essential for maintaining a healthy herbal garden. Embrace organic gardening practices by using natural fertilizers and avoiding synthetic pesticides. Pay attention to signs of pests or diseases and address them promptly using eco-friendly methods.

Harvesting and Drying:

Harvest your herbs when they are at their peak potency, usually in the morning after the dew has dried. Use sharp scissors or pruners to avoid damaging the plants. To dry your herbs, hang them in bundles in a warm, well-ventilated area away from direct sunlight. Once dry, store them in airtight containers away from heat and moisture.

Creating a Healing Sanctuary:

Transform your herbal garden into a sanctuary of healing by adding elements like comfortable seating, soothing water features, and aromatic plants. Take time to connect with your garden, whether it's through meditation, journaling, or simply enjoying the sights and scents.

By embracing the art of growing your own medicinal herbs, you not only reap the physical benefits of herbal remedies but also nourish your soul and deepen your connection to the natural world. Let your herbal garden be a reflection of your commitment to health, sustainability, and holistic well-being.

Unlock the healing potential of common herbs for everyday health concerns. From soothing chamomile for stress relief to potent garlic for immune support, discover the versatility of nature's pharmacy. Explore herbal remedies for headaches, digestion, sleep, and more, empowering yourself to take charge of your well-being naturally.

Herbs have been used for centuries to address a wide range of health concerns. Here are some common herbs and their healing potential for everyday health issues:

1. **Chamomile**: Known for its calming properties, chamomile can help relieve stress and anxiety. It's also beneficial for promoting better sleep and soothing upset stomachs.

2. **Peppermint**: Peppermint is excellent for digestive issues such as bloating, indigestion, and nausea. It can also provide relief from tension headaches when applied topically or inhaled as an essential oil.

3. **Ginger**: Ginger is well-known for its ability to alleviate nausea and aid digestion. It can also help reduce inflammation and relieve muscle pain.

4. **Lavender**: Lavender is renowned for its calming scent, which can help reduce stress and promote relaxation. It's often used in aromatherapy to improve sleep quality and alleviate headaches.

5. **Echinacea**: Echinacea is commonly used to support the immune system and reduce the severity and duration of colds and flu. It can also help alleviate symptoms of respiratory infections.

6. **Eucalyptus**: Eucalyptus is excellent for relieving congestion and promoting clearer breathing. It's often used in steam inhalations or as an ingredient in chest rubs for coughs and colds.

7. **Valerian**: Valerian root is a natural sedative that can help improve sleep quality and alleviate insomnia. It's often used in herbal teas or supplements for its calming effects.

8. **Turmeric**: Turmeric contains curcumin, a compound with powerful anti-inflammatory and antioxidant properties. It can help reduce inflammation, relieve joint pain, and support overall health.

9. **Garlic**: Garlic is well-known for its immune-boosting properties. It can help fight off infections, reduce the severity of colds, and support cardiovascular health.

10. **Lemon Balm**: Lemon balm has calming effects and can help reduce stress and anxiety. It's also beneficial for promoting better sleep and easing digestive discomfort.

These herbs can be used in various forms, including teas, tinctures, capsules, essential oils, and as fresh or dried ingredients in cooking. However, it's essential to consult with a healthcare professional before using herbal remedies, especially if you have any underlying health conditions or are taking medications.

Chapter 5: Herbs for mind, body and spirit

Journey deeper into the holistic realm of herbal medicine, exploring the connections between physical health, emotional balance, and spiritual well-being. Discover herbs that uplift the mood, calm the mind, and nourish the soul. From adaptogens to nervines, explore the herbs that support resilience and promote inner harmony.

Embarking on a journey into the holistic realm of herbal medicine is an enriching path that intertwines the realms of physical health, emotional balance, and spiritual well-being. Herbs have been revered for centuries for their multifaceted healing properties, which extend beyond mere physical ailments to encompass the intricate web of mind, body, and spirit.

Adaptogens: These remarkable herbs possess the unique ability to support the body's resilience to stress, promoting balance and vitality. Adaptogens like ashwagandha, holy basil (Tulsi), and rhodiola rosea help the body adapt to various stressors, both internal and external, thereby fostering a sense of equilibrium amidst life's challenges. Incorporating adaptogens into your routine can enhance overall well-being and promote emotional stability.

Nervines: Nervines are herbs that have a calming and soothing effect on the nervous system, offering relief from anxiety, tension, and restlessness. Chamomile, passionflower, and lemon balm are renowned nervines that promote relaxation and tranquility, easing the mind and facilitating a deeper sense of calm. These herbs can be particularly beneficial for those experiencing stress-related symptoms or struggling with sleep disturbances.

Mood Uplifters: Certain herbs possess uplifting properties that can elevate mood and foster a sense of joy and optimism. St. John's Wort, known for its antidepressant effects, is often used to alleviate symptoms of mild to moderate depression and seasonal affective disorder (SAD). Additionally, herbs like rosemary, lavender, and damiana have mood-enhancing qualities that can brighten the spirit and promote emotional well-being.

Soul-Nourishing Herbs: Beyond their physical and emotional benefits, some herbs are revered for their profound spiritual significance and soul-nourishing qualities. Plants like sage, palo santo, and cedar are used in rituals and ceremonies to purify energy, offer protection, and cultivate spiritual connection. Incorporating these sacred herbs into your spiritual practices can facilitate inner exploration, deepen meditation, and enhance mindfulness.

Herbal Rituals and Practices: Engaging in herbal rituals and practices can deepen your connection to the plant kingdom and amplify the healing benefits of herbs. Whether it's brewing a cup of herbal tea mindfully, incorporating herbs into your bath or skincare routine, or creating sacred herbal bundles for smudging ceremonies, these rituals can become sacred moments of self-care and introspection.

As you journey deeper into the holistic realm of herbal medicine, remember to approach herbs with reverence, mindfulness, and gratitude for their profound healing gifts. By embracing the interconnectedness of physical health, emotional balance, and spiritual well-being, you can cultivate a harmonious relationship with nature and experience profound transformation on all levels of being.

Chapter 6: Harvesting herbs for sustainability

Harvesting herbs sustainably is crucial for preserving their populations and ensuring their availability for future generations. Here's a guide to proper harvesting:

1. **Know Your Herbs**: Understand the growth habits, life cycles, and specific needs of the herbs you're harvesting. Different herbs require different harvesting techniques and timing.

2. **Harvest Responsibly**: Only harvest from abundant populations of herbs. Avoid harvesting rare or endangered species, and never take more than what you need.

3. **Timing**: Harvest herbs at the right time to maximize flavor and potency. Generally, it's best to harvest herbs early in the morning after the dew has dried but before the sun is too strong. This is when their essential oils are most concentrated.

4. **Selective Harvesting**: Rather than harvesting entire plants, selectively pick leaves, flowers, or seeds. This allows the plant to continue growing and producing more foliage.

5. **Use Sharp Tools**: Use sharp, clean scissors or pruning shears to make clean cuts. Avoid tearing or damaging the plant, as this can lead to infection or slow regrowth.

6. **Leave Some Behind**: Leave some herbs behind to ensure the plant's survival and allow it to produce seeds for future growth.

7. **Rotate Harvesting Areas**: If you're harvesting from wild populations, rotate harvesting areas to allow plants to recover and prevent depletion of resources in a single area.

8. **Sustainable Cultivation**: Consider growing your own herbs in a garden or container. This allows you to control growing conditions and ensures a sustainable supply.

9. **Support Local Growers**: Purchase herbs from local farmers or growers who practice sustainable harvesting methods. This supports local economies and encourages responsible stewardship of the land.

10. **Learn Preservation Techniques**: Learn how to preserve herbs through drying, freezing, or making herbal extracts. Properly preserved herbs can be enjoyed throughout the year without the need for continuous harvesting.

By following these guidelines, you can enjoy the benefits of fresh herbs while promoting their sustainability for future generations.

Delving into the world of herbal remedies is a wonderful journey! Here's a comprehensive guide to help you master the art of preparing herbal remedies at home:

Getting Started:

1. **Research**: Begin by researching different herbs, their properties, and potential uses. Books, reputable websites, and even local herbalists can be valuable resources.

2. **Safety First**: Understand the safety considerations and potential interactions of herbs, especially if you're using them for medicinal purposes. Some herbs can interact with medications or have side effects.

3. **Sourcing Herbs**: Choose high-quality, organic herbs whenever possible. You can grow your own herbs or purchase them from reputable suppliers.

Basic Herbal Preparations:

1. **Herbal Infusions (Teas)**:

   - Infusions involve steeping herbs in hot water to extract their medicinal properties. Adjust the strength by varying the herb-to-water ratio and steeping time.

   - Example: Chamomile tea for relaxation or peppermint tea for digestion.

2. **Herbal Decoctions**:

  - Decoctions are similar to infusions but involve boiling tougher
plant parts like roots, bark, or seeds to extract their constituents.

  - Example: Astragalus root decoction for immune support.

3. **Herbal Tinctures**:

  - Tinctures are concentrated liquid extracts made by steeping
herbs in alcohol or glycerin. They have a longer shelf life and are
convenient for dosage control.

  - Example: Echinacea tincture for immune support.

4. **Herbal Oils**:

  - Infuse herbs into carrier oils (like olive or coconut oil) to create
herbal oils for massage, skincare, or culinary purposes.

  - Example: Lavender-infused oil for relaxation or calendula-
infused oil for skin healing.

5. **Herbal Salves and Balms**:

  - Combine herbal-infused oils with beeswax to create healing
salves or balms for topical application.

  - Example: Calendula salve for soothing minor skin irritations.

6. **Herbal Syrups**:

  - Make herbal syrups by simmering herbs with water and
sweeteners like honey or sugar. These are great for respiratory
support or soothing sore throats.

  - Example: Elderberry syrup for immune support during cold and
flu season.

Techniques:

1. **Harvesting and Drying Herbs**: Harvest herbs at the right time, typically when they're in full bloom, and dry them properly to preserve their potency.

2. **Extraction Methods**: Experiment with different extraction methods like maceration, percolation, or enfleurage to extract specific constituents from herbs.

3. **Dosage and Storage**: Keep track of dosages and store your herbal remedies properly in a cool, dark place to maintain their efficacy.

Recipes:

Elderberry syrup with honey:

Ingredients:

- 1 cup dried elderberries

- 4 cups water

- 1 cup honey (preferably raw or local)

Instructions:

1. **Prepare the elderberries**: Rinse the dried elderberries under cold water to remove any debris.

2. **Boil the elderberries**: In a saucepan, combine the elderberries and water. Bring the mixture to a boil, then reduce the heat to low and let it simmer for about 30-45 minutes, or until the liquid is reduced by half.

3. **Strain the mixture**: Once the mixture has simmered and reduced, remove it from the heat and let it cool slightly. Strain the liquid through a fine mesh sieve or cheesecloth into a clean bowl or jar, pressing down on the berries to extract as much liquid as possible. Discard the elderberry solids.

4. **Add honey**: Let the elderberry liquid cool to lukewarm temperature, then stir in the honey until it's completely dissolved.

5. **Store the syrup**: Transfer the elderberry syrup to a clean, airtight container, such as a glass jar or bottle. Store it in the refrigerator for up to 2-3 months.

Usage:

- Take 1-2 tablespoons daily as a preventative measure during cold and flu season.

- If you feel a cold or flu coming on, you can increase the dosage to 1-2 tablespoons every 2-3 hours until symptoms improve.

Enjoy your homemade elderberry syrup!

Calendula salve:

Ingredients:

- 1 cup dried calendula petals

- 1 cup carrier oil (such as olive oil, coconut oil, or almond oil)

- 2 tablespoons beeswax pellets

Instructions:

1. **Infuse the oil**: In a clean, dry glass jar, combine the dried calendula petals and the carrier oil of your choice. Make sure the petals are fully submerged in the oil. Seal the jar tightly and place it in a warm, sunny spot for about 4-6 weeks to infuse. Alternatively, you can use a double boiler to gently heat the mixture for 2-3 hours, but the solar infusion method tends to retain more of the plant's beneficial properties.

2. **Strain the oil**: After the infusion period, strain the oil through a fine mesh sieve or cheesecloth into a clean, dry bowl or saucepan to remove the calendula petals. Squeeze out as much oil from the petals as possible.

3. **Melt the beeswax**: In a double boiler or a heatproof bowl set over a pot of simmering water, melt the beeswax pellets.

4. **Combine the ingredients**: Once the beeswax is completely melted, slowly pour in the infused calendula oil while stirring continuously. Stir until the mixture is well combined and smooth.

5. **Test the consistency**: To test the consistency of the salve, you can place a small amount on a spoon and let it cool for a few seconds. If it's too soft, add more beeswax. If it's too firm, add more infused oil.

6. **Pour into containers**: Once you've reached the desired consistency, carefully pour the mixture into clean, dry containers, such as jars or tins. Allow the salve to cool completely before sealing the containers with lids.

7. **Label and store**: Label your calendula salve with the date it was made and any other relevant information. Store it in a cool, dark place away from direct sunlight.

Usage:

- Apply the calendula salve to dry or irritated skin as needed.

- It can also be used as a soothing balm for minor cuts, scrapes, and insect bites.

Peppermint Tea

Ingredients:

- Fresh peppermint leaves or dried peppermint leaves

- Water

Instructions:

1. **Prepare the peppermint leaves**: If you're using fresh peppermint leaves, rinse them thoroughly under cold water to remove any dirt or debris. If you're using dried peppermint leaves, you can skip this step.

2. **Boil water**: In a pot or kettle, bring water to a boil. You'll need about 1 cup of water for each serving of tea.

3. **Steep the peppermint leaves**: Place about 1 tablespoon of fresh peppermint leaves or 1 teaspoon of dried peppermint leaves into a teapot or a heatproof mug.

4. **Pour the hot water**: Once the water has reached a rolling boil, carefully pour it over the peppermint leaves in the teapot or mug.

5. **Steep the tea**: Cover the teapot or mug with a lid or a small plate to trap the heat and let the peppermint leaves steep in the hot water for about 5-10 minutes. The longer you steep the tea, the stronger the flavor will be.

6. **Strain (optional)**: If you used loose peppermint leaves, you may want to strain the tea before serving to remove the leaves. You can use a fine mesh sieve or a tea strainer for this.

7. **Serve**: Pour the peppermint tea into cups and enjoy it hot. You can sweeten it with honey or sugar if desired, or enjoy it as it is.

Variations:

- For a refreshing twist, you can add a slice of lemon or a sprig of fresh mint to your peppermint tea.

- You can also chill the tea in the refrigerator after steeping to make a refreshing iced peppermint tea.

Peppermint tea is not only delicious but also has potential health benefits, such as aiding digestion and providing relief from headaches or nausea. Enjoy your homemade peppermint tea!

Arnica Salve

Arnica salve is commonly used for its potential anti-inflammatory and pain-relieving properties. Here's a basic recipe to make your own:

Ingredients:

- 1 cup carrier oil (such as olive oil, coconut oil, or almond oil)

- 1/4 cup dried arnica flowers

- 2 tablespoons beeswax pellets

Instructions:

1. **Infuse the oil**: In a clean, dry glass jar, combine the dried arnica flowers and the carrier oil of your choice. Ensure the flowers are fully submerged in the oil. Seal the jar tightly and place it in a warm, sunny spot for about 4-6 weeks to infuse. Alternatively, you can use a double boiler to gently heat the mixture for 2-3 hours.

2. **Strain the oil**: After the infusion period, strain the oil through a fine mesh sieve or cheesecloth into a clean, dry bowl or saucepan to remove the arnica flowers. Squeeze out as much oil from the flowers as possible.

3. **Melt the beeswax**: In a double boiler or a heatproof bowl set over a pot of simmering water, melt the beeswax pellets.

4. **Combine the ingredients**: Once the beeswax is completely melted, slowly pour in the infused arnica oil while stirring continuously. Stir until the mixture is well combined and smooth.

5. **Test the consistency**: To test the consistency of the salve, you can place a small amount on a spoon and let it cool for a few seconds. If it's too soft, add more beeswax. If it's too firm, add more infused oil.

6. **Pour into containers**: Once you've reached the desired consistency, carefully pour the mixture into clean, dry containers, such as jars or tins. Allow the salve to cool completely before sealing the containers with lids.

7. **Label and store**: Label your arnica salve with the date it was made and any other relevant information. Store it in a cool, dark place away from direct sunlight.

Usage:

- Apply the arnica salve to areas of soreness, bruises, or minor injuries as needed.

- Avoid using arnica salve on broken skin or open wounds, and discontinue use if any irritation occurs.

Remember that while arnica salve is popular for its potential benefits, it's always a good idea to consult with a healthcare professional before using it, especially if you have any underlying health conditions or are pregnant or breastfeeding.

Anti Cough Medicine

Here's a simple recipe for a natural cough medicine using common ingredients:

Ingredients:

- 1 cup honey (preferably raw or local)

- 1 medium-sized lemon

- 2-3 inches of fresh ginger root

- Optional: 1-2 cloves of garlic, finely minced

Instructions:

1. **Prepare the ingredients**: Wash the lemon and ginger root thoroughly. Slice the lemon into thin rounds. Peel the ginger root and slice it into thin rounds or grate it finely. If using garlic, peel and finely mince it.

2. **Combine the ingredients**: In a clean, dry glass jar with a lid, layer the lemon slices and ginger slices (and minced garlic, if using) until the jar is about halfway full. Pour the honey over the lemon and ginger until they are completely covered.

3. **Infuse the mixture**: Seal the jar tightly and let it sit at room temperature for at least 24 hours, but preferably 2-3 days. During this time, the honey will slowly infuse with the flavors of the lemon and ginger.

4. **Strain (optional)**: After the infusion period, you can strain the mixture through a fine mesh sieve or cheesecloth to remove

the lemon and ginger pieces, leaving you with a smooth cough syrup. Alternatively, you can leave the pieces in the honey for added flavor and texture.

5. **Store the cough syrup**: Transfer the strained or unstrained cough syrup to a clean, airtight container, such as a glass jar or bottle. Store it in the refrigerator for up to 1-2 months.

Usage:

- Take 1-2 teaspoons of the cough syrup as needed to soothe coughs and sore throats. You can take it straight off the spoon or mix it into a cup of warm water or herbal tea.

- Be aware that honey should not be given to infants under one year of age due to the risk of botulism.

This natural cough medicine combines the soothing properties of honey, lemon, and ginger, and the optional addition of garlic can provide additional immune support. However, if your cough persists or worsens, it's essential to consult with a healthcare professional for proper diagnosis and treatment.

Remember, herbal remedies can be powerful allies in supporting health and wellness, but it's essential to consult with a healthcare professional, especially if you have any pre-existing health conditions or are pregnant or breastfeeding. Enjoy your herbal journey!

Conclusion: Embracing the Healing Wisdom of Nature

As we journey through the pages of "Healing Earth: A Guide to Medicinal Herbs," we come to realize that the path to wellness is intertwined with the natural world. By embracing the healing wisdom of nature, we honor the interconnectedness of all living beings and cultivate a deeper relationship with the earth. May this book serve as a guide and a companion on your journey to health, vitality, and wholeness.